How I Gave Up Sugar and Took Control of My Diet in 7 Days

From the popular website
TheSugarFreeDiva.com

Annie Busco
The Sugar Free Diva

This book Is dedicated to everyone in my life who has respected my decisions, supported those decisions, and has not attempted to sabotage those decisions. I am lucky to have been able to enjoy the sweet life anyway as a result.

1st Edition

Copyright

Disclaimer - this book is intended to be for reference and entertainment. It is not intended to be for use as a nutritional, dietary, or other kind of guideline. The author is not a dietician nor a doctor and takes no responsibility for the results that come from reader actions. Please consult a professional.

Introduction

While planning this book my goals were to both share my journey for a sugar free lifestyle and help motivate others with their journey.

While it may not be for you, I am hopeful that my journey may help motivate you in reaching your own sugar related goals. Giving up sugar can be hard to do. However, you are not alone in the journey.

Before we begin, there are a few concepts that I would like to share with you. You will see references to these concepts throughout this book.

First of all, this book, as well as my other books and my website, are not intended to be targeted at or a bashing of the sugar industry. Nor is this book intended to be an endorsement of any specific sugar alternative(s).

Also, this book is not intended to be a diet book. I am not a dietician or a physician. If you are looking to lose weight by controlling your sugar intake, obviously you should seek medical advice first, just as with any diet.

My personal sugar journey is quite simple. I did not like the way the sugar that I consumed in my diet controlled me. As a result, I sought to control that sugar instead of it controlling me. I started out totally sugar free and have since evolved to consuming only the sugar that comes from fresh fruit.

I am not totally sugar free at this specific moment. Rather, I am sugar controlled. This is what works for me and my life. I feel great physically and mentally as well.

This method for controlling the sugar in my life is what works for me.

This book is divided into three sections. The first section is about my motivation and the research that led me to my decision to break up with sugar.

The second section focuses on my sugar free challenge. This was the week that I broke up with sugar. I share how I did it and the skills that I focused on each day.

The remainder of this book focuses on living a sugar free lifestyle beyond the sugar free challenge. Once I broke up with sugar I had to learn how to live without it.

Section 1:My Motivation

I am a 'reformed sugar addict'

What exactly is a 'reformed sugar addict'?

Let me begin with my personal journey. This is the story about how sugar took over my life and what I did about it. To be honest, it wasn't until I hit the 'brick wall' that I realized there was a problem. It was the brick wall that was my motivation.

My sugar journey began in my childhood, as I am sure yours might have begun as well. In those days, there really was no 'sugar free movement'. We certainly have evolved since those days in so many ways.

I can trace my earliest 'romance' with sugar to the punch that my mother would serve me to drink when I was in grade school. I will not say the particular name of the brand of punch but, I will mention that it came in a large can and suburban moms were convinced by great marketing tactics that it was a must-have in every refrigerator in America. Thus, it was always readily available to me as a kid.

That punch was loaded with both sugar and a certain red dye that was later proven to be harmful. I will focus on the sugar in that punch right now. The dye is a whole other book idea that is not for me to investigate at this time.

My sugar addiction, via this red punch, is like so many other sugar addiction stories. It started with a glass and moved on to a 'gotta have more of it' feeling. Like many addictions, you start small and constantly want more. The more you enjoy, the more that you need to have.

Obviously, my body was affected by all of that sugar. After drinking the punch, I would become a hyperactive and often uncontrollable kid all thanks to that sugar high. That hyperactive feeling would be followed by that sleepy sluggish drop in energy. I call this the 'sugar rollercoaster'.

I hit that brick wall when I realized how sugar in my life became an endless cycle. The more that I ate or drank, the more that I craved. The more that I craved, the more that I ate or drank. The sugar was controlling me. I was not controlling it.

I wish that I could say that the sugar cycle never caused me any physical problems. However, it did. My sugar addiction certainly gave me challenges with my body weight . Eating a lot of sugar made me lazy as the sugar lows made me sluggish. To this day I am plagued with reminders thanks to the dental problems that still affect me.

Unfortunately, I did not realize that sugar was doing all of this to me until I became an adult. It seems that often it is when we become an adult that we realize that we are responsible for our behavior. Realizing that sugar was responsible for my behavior was my 'light bulb moment'. I refer to this as the time when I hit 'my sugar brick wall'.

For me it was certainly the sugar in that punch that started my sugar problem. After I got use to the punch I moved on to the candy from the local drug store and sweet treats when I would venture out to other places.

This book takes you on the journey that I took as an adult, after I hit the brick wall. It is how I had finally had enough of the sugar roller coaster and decided to do something about it. I am really glad that I took this course in life as I am feeling better about myself as a result.I got tired of sugar controlling me physically and mentally.

I decided to 'reform' my sugar addiction.

Reforming meant controlling sugar rather than sugar controlling me. I had enough of the sugar rollercoaster cycle.

What worked for me was to first challenge myself to give up sugar. I decided that I would start the challenge with a weeklong effort to rid the sugar in my life. This effort would clear out the sugar in my life in order to successfully move on with my taking control of the sugar in my life forever.

The start of controlling the sugar in my life that had been controlling me.

The anger at my sugar problem was the motivation that I needed to get rid of it from my life. The first week of giving up sugar is what I would refer to my 'cold turkey week'. I got rid of the sugar in my life in one week. That week taught me that I could be successful in taking control.

The 'cold turkey week' is a rather structured week. It would have to be to keep me focused and inline rather than straying and giving up. I decided to set goals and structure to the week.

Each day of my 'cold turkey week' focused on an aspect of taking sugar control that needed attention. Each aspect was something that needed to be tackled in order to reach my goal of dealing with my sugar addiction. I will explain this in better detail in coming chapters.

My 'cold turkey week' became my challenge.

Certainly gaining control of sugar was my biggest challenge. However, to do this I needed a week long challenge of a 'cold turkey week' to get me started.

Why did I need a week long aka 'cold turkey week? Well, certainly to 'kick my butt' for starters. The reality was that I needed a plan in the form of a challenge because simply cutting back of sugar was something that would not work for me. It is just too easy to fail when there is no structured plan.

Simply cutting back on something, rather than having a structured plan, never seems to work well . Not having a plan can make it too easy to fail when there is temptation. Even worse, sometimes, it creeps back even more than it was before cutting back.

Taking seven days allowed me to focus on everything that made me want more sugar while giving me the satisfaction of success for doing so. Each day of my seven day challenge I was motivated by what I had successfully tackled the day before. It all started when I defined what my ultimate 'giving up sugar' goal actually was.

Defining what 'giving up sugar' is an important step to start with.

I do have my own definition of 'giving up sugar'. My definition of giving up sugar means giving up all of those foods which have had sugar added to them. My definition of giving up sugar means that

I eat the natural sugar (fruit) in moderation. When I bake, I use the sugar alternatives. My definition is what works for me just as your definition is what works for you.

As I have mentioned, while my sugar free journey may not be for you, it may inspire you in some way. It is important to do what is best for you.

I will mention that I have never been diagnosed as a diabetic nor am I an expert on the issue. I am just sharing what has worked for me.

I am going to touch on sugar alternatives rather than go into depth about them.

If you are interested in learning more about sugar alternatives, check out my Guide for Baking with Sugar Alternatives, which is available on Amazon.

How to use this guide

As I have mentioned, to start my sugar free journey, I went on a seven day challenge. This guide chronicles how I did that challenge.

Seven days is obviously a week. It took me a week to give up sugar. Before I embarked on that week, I started with a bit of preparation as I will explain.

Before we begin, I will tell you that this guide is not intended to be a 'bash-fest' on sugar or the sugar industry. Nor is this guide intended to serve as a diet book.
Those would be too easy to do. Instead, this guide is more of a re-thinking and updating of a lifestyle. A lifestyle where sugar is controlled rather than being the controller.

So let's start by talking about sugar.

About that Sugar
I gave up sugar because I did not like how I felt after eating it.

Sugar puts me on a rollercoaster.
I never liked being on that rollercoaster. The rollercoaster of the sugar highs that is followed to the sugar lows. One minute I have a lot of energy and a short while later I need a nap.

It is not just the sugar rollercoaster that turned me into a sugar free person. Sugar consumption took its toll on my weight as well as my teeth. In the end, I always felt controlled by sugar rather than me controlling the sugar.

There seems to be a lot of research out there about sugar.

I actually never paid a lot of attention to all of that research until after I made my life change from sugar controlled to sugar controller. The research just reinforced my decision. Giving up sugar is what has worked for me.

Sugar consumption, like tobacco, eating beef or pork, sunbathing, wrestling with alligators, is a personal thing. If it works for you or is something that you want to do, you will probably do it.

The Research on Sugar

Here is some of the research that I took into consideration when I decided to control the sugar in my life.

Sugar, according to the National Institute of Health (NIH), is "a functional ingredient for baking, texturizing, and preserving". It comes naturally in foods such as fruit and dairy. The NIH says that majority of sugar in the US diet is added to processed food and beverages" This added sugar is often added to enhance the taste of something rather than serving as a texturized or preserver. That added sugar is what I had to take control over.

The fact that a majority of sugar that we consume did not get into what we are eating naturally, can be of some concern to many of us. I know that this added sugar has affected many of my food choices.

However, the good news is that we Americans are getting smarter about the sugar that we are consuming.

Have you noticed a recent influx of beverages that are not sugared sodas and that are actually variations of water? I have. There is a reason why we are seeing less of the sugared sodas and more of the water based beverages.The reason is that manufacturers are listening to what consumers are saying.

As consumers we have spoken via our purchasing power and many manufacturers have listened . The result is less sugar in our beverages.

Getting back to the discussion of sugar, the NIH says that there are reasons to want to cut back on sugar.

• Sugar consumptions adds to weight gain. You probably already know this. There are actual studies that link weight gain to the sugar that is added to beverages and food we consumer.

•About those products with the added sugar. The added sugar usually just provides with calories but, no additional nutrients. So basically all that you are getting from consuming that added sugar is a sweeter taste and possibly a few negative results such as weight gain.

You may also have heard about these health concerns as well.

The American Heart Association says that weight gain over the past 30 years in the United States "must be related in part to increased intake of added sugars," which also "appears to be associated with increased triglyceride levels, a known risk factor for coronary heart disease."

At this point you may be asking yourself what amount of sugar is okay to eat.

What is the recommended daily intake of sugar anyway? Some sugar consumption could be acceptable, up to a point.

The folks who give us advice about how to take care of our hearts (American Heart Association-AHA) recommend this:

> **"Limiting the amount of added sugars you consume to no more than half of your daily discretionary calories allowance. For most American women, that's no more than 100 calories per day, or about 6 teaspoons of sugar. For men, it's 150 calories per day, or about 9 teaspoons."**

How does that AHA recommendation compare to real life?

I am mentioning this because of the link between obesity and sugar as well as the prevalence of prepared foods available today. Some of the following tidbits still amaze me as I read them over and over.

•Before there were grocery stores with prepared food (over 100 years ago basically), American's consumed about 2 pounds of sugar in a year. 2 pounds is about 192 teaspoons which would mean that Americans consumed about half a teaspoon of sugar in a day. Wow!

•50 years ago (about the time of the onset of suburbia and grocery stores) that amount of consumed sugar jumped up to over 120 pounds of sugar in a year. 11,520 teaspoons or 31 1/2 teaspoons of sugar per day.

•Today American's have decreased their consumption of sugar to as much as 20+ teaspoons of sugar daily (according to the AHA). Education and smart consumer choices have made an impact on sugar consumption according to the experts. Hence, the prior discussion about consumer demands for more of the healthy water beverages.

Here is the scoop on sugar.

•One teaspoon of white sugar has about 15 calories in it.

•One teaspoon of corn syrup has about 20 calories in it. I am mentioning this because many soft drinks are sweetened with corn syrup and not sugar per se. There could be over 10 teaspoons of corn syrup in one can of soda as a result! That's 200 calories just from corn syrup in that can of soda.

•There is a recommended amount of sugar that Americans should consume according to AHA and other experts. They say that 10% of our calories should come from sugar.

•Based on a 2000 calories diet, we should consume 13.3 teaspoons of sugar per day. Of course, this may not be for everyone and you should consult your professional to see what is best for you.

And then there are those hidden sugars.

As they say in this social media society, OMG!

I have become one of those crazy label reading people as I have gotten older. I cannot believe where I find sugar.

Medicine, such as cough syrup, can contain sugar. Breath mints can have sugar. Sauces, cereals, 'healthy' bars, dressings, sauces, ketchup, yogurt, peanut butter, drink mixes, canned and preserved food, and even chewing gum have it too

How to find the sugar in what you eat and drink.

As a restaurant owner, I can tell you that there are regulations concerning restaurants providing nutritional information to people. As consumers, we are privy to nutritional information on what we purchase, thanks to rules.

There is a reason why this information is readily available. It is because there may be something important that we need to know about when it comes to the food that we eat.

The information that is on the label informs us on what we need to know in order to take care of ourselves. If we are sensitive to sugar, we need to be aware of the sugar that we consume.

Reading the label on the foods and beverages that we consume help us determine if there is sugar in what we eat and drink.

By the way, while there may not necessarily be a 'good sugar' there are natural sugars as opposed to manufactured ones. For some, simply giving up the added processed sugar is fine. For others, controlling all and any sugar is what is needed.

When you read food labels, you may want to look for these names for sugar:

- Sucrose (table sugar)
- High-fructose corn syrup
- Molasses
- Glucose
- Fructose
- Fruit juice concentrates
- Honey
- Sugar
- Maltose
- Corn sweetener
- Syrup, corn, rice, etc
- Malt
- Sucrose
- Dextrose, anhydrous dextrose, crystal dextrose

As you can tell, there are many different names for sugar. That is because there are so many different kinds of sugar. I have only listed a portion of them.

This means that there are many different sugars to have to look out for as a result. Learning about the different kinds of sugars can help you make helpful decisions about what you eat.

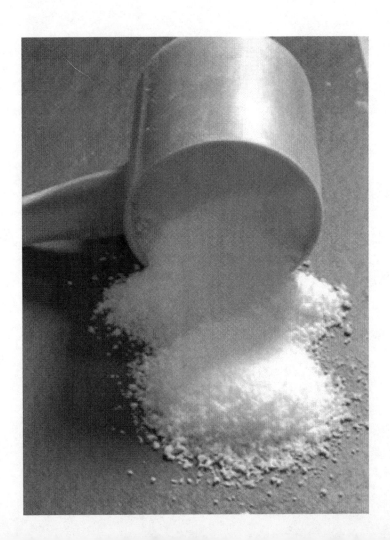

You may be wondering about the use of natural sugar such as what is in honey or molasses.

While these both honey and molasses do contain sugar, there are people who will use either of the two as a sugar alternative. I know people who eat honey because of research concerning the health benefits of doing so.

In the case of molasses, it has a slower affect on blood sugar which makes it friendlier for some diabetics. I personally consider both to be 'sugar' as they do contain sugar in them.

However, I have also used honey and molasses in moderation while baking. This was not necessarily for sweetening purposes.

This guide offers a seven day sugar free challenge.

You want to make a change but, you are not sure how to get it started. That was how I felt. I decided to start with a self challenge.

I kicked off my sugar free lifestyle with a seven day challenge. as I have mentioned in this book. Now, I will go further into depth about this challenge.

The challenge is something that I did. However, you do not have to follow the challenge. You may even choose to follow part of the challenge.

The following chapters focus on each of the seven days of my seven day challenge. Within each challenge day there is a focus for the day, a goal for the day and the big change of the day. The focus, goal, and change for each day is offered as a suggestion and for motivational purposes.

We all know that giving up sugar can be difficult especially at first. However, knowing that others have gone through it too can be helpful. You may or may not be thinking or feeling what I mention for each day. Every seven day challenge or journey can differ.

The seven day challenge is meant to be a tool that may help you too.

Following the challenge, the remainder of this book focuses on maintaining that sugar free lifestyle. Learning how to live without sugar would seem to be the likely thing to do after giving it up.

Learning how to control sugar can mean going sugar free or going sugar controlled.

The difference between being sugar free and sugar controlled would be that one omits all and any sugar while the other accepts sugar in moderation.

In this guide, both sugar free and sugar controlled may be referred to as 'sugar free'. For the purposes of this guide, "sugar free" can also mean low or controlled sugar. Please do not get caught up in the terminology and refer to the definition of sugar free that suits your needs.

We will begin with the seven day sugar free challenge because this is a way to get into both the sugar free mindset and the sugar free lifestyle. Both concepts work together when it comes to reaching our goals.

While you may not want to follow the challenge itself, you may find that parts of it may be worth trying. I suggest doing what works best for you, your goals, and your situation.

To sum up this chapter, I have so far given you my argument about why I have decided to rid my lifestyle of sugar. I have also given you information about sugar and how it affects us, as per the experts and the research. Lastly, you have been introduced to the concepts of this book and the sugar free challenge weeklong kickoff.

In the next chapter we will discuss the seven day sugar free challenge.

Section 2: The Sugar Free Challenge

The beginning of a new way of eating.

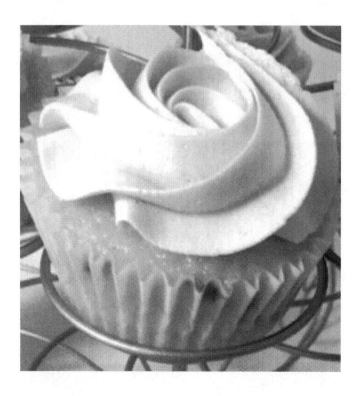

You have read the argument for why we could consider cutting out sugar. Now we can prepare to do just so.

Preparation is really the key factor to success when it comes to taking on something that can change our lifestyle like this can. There is a lot to prepare for when it comes to a lifestyle change after all.

Preparing to get rid of sugar.

As mentioned, preparation is what we will do before we actually start that week without sugar. It is the preparation that will help up identify a purpose, a path, and a goal. Since this is a seven day journey, I will also call it a week.

As I have mentioned in the last chapter, following through with the seven day sugar free challenge is certainly optional. However, I think that reading the chapter is essential. This is because there are strategies that may help you begin your sugar free journey even without a challenge.

Let's start by mapping out the week. We will start mapping out the week by identifying our motivation and goals. Then we will decide just what 'sugar free' means followed by some sugar housecleaning. Lastly, we will prepare for that week of going without sugar.

Here are the four steps that you can do to help you prepare for going sugar free.*

Step one: identify your sugar free goals and motivations. Ask yourself these questions.

‣ Why are you going sugar free?

‣ Will this be a permanent lifestyle change?

‣ Are you 100% behind doing this?

‣ What is the intended result from going without sugar?

‣ How will you measure your intended result success?

Step two: Next, decide if you will be going totally sugar free or if you would like to be 'sugar controlled'.

‣ Sugar free as in no sugar what so ever.

‣ Sugar controlled as in no refined or added sugar.

‣ Sugar controlled as in only natural sugar.

‣ Sugar Controlled as in just eat less of the stuff.

Step three: Clean out the sugar from the kitchen, office, everywhere else.

▸ Clean out the sugar from your cupboards, drawers, etc. Anything that will tempt you in the next week and thus, set you up for failure, get rid of it.

▸ Get rid of any food that contains sugar as well as the sugar itself.

Step four: Prepare or shop for new food.

Shopping List.

▸ Sugar free beverages- water, tea, soda etc.

▸ Sugar alternatives- sweeteners that are not sugar.

▸ Sugar free dressings, sauces, jams, etc.

▸ Replacement foods (fruit, vegetables, other)

▸ Diversion food- sugar free mints etc.

Step five: Optional, The last hoorah.

The last thing that I did before I started was to get sugar out of my system. I allowed sugar to get into my system one last time.

This step may not be for you. I more or less overdosed on sugar to the point that I was done and never wanted to eat it ever again. In the end, I was ready to start my week of going sugar free.

Is this for you too? That is for you to decide.

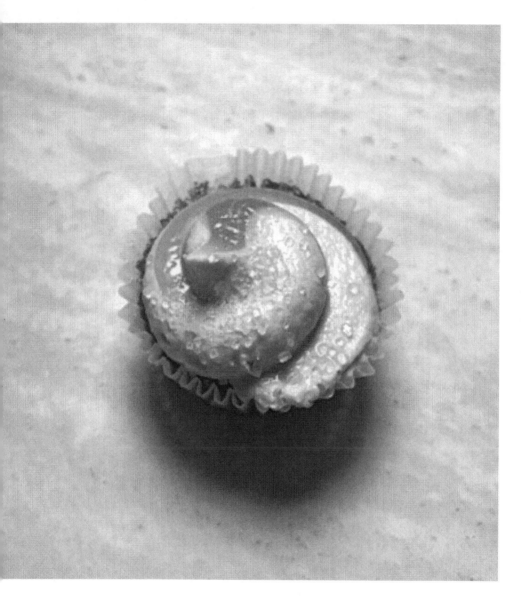

About the sugar free challenge.

I am starting this out with an overview of the sugar free challenge. Then I will focus on the specifics.

Each day in the seven day challenge has three points that we will touch upon. The first point will be the goal of the day. Each day will also have its own focus as well as the change that results from the points of that day.

- **Goal(s)-** The goals are the desired results from that day of the challenge. One goal will be the big goal of the day.

- **Focus-** A daily focus is an action or idea that will give us something to think about.

- **Change-** What change will result from that day of the challenge.A change can be due to our focus and can help achieve our goals.

One of our daily goals will be our most important goal of the day. I will call that the big goal of the day.

This big goal of the day may be confusing to you right now. The big goal can have smaller goals that lead up to it. For example, your big goal of the day may be to become more active. Another goal may be what you want to do to become more active. Perhaps, taking a 20 minute walk and a 10 minute stretch are two goals that you may take toward that one big goal of becoming more active.

Think of those smaller goals as objectives if that makes it clearer for you to understand. However, since these smaller goals may also lead to lifestyle changes, I like to refer to them as goals as well. Those smaller goals help to lead us to that one big goal of the day.

The focus of the day is more of a psychological motivation rather than just a physical one. We all know the importance of the mind when it comes to making a lifestyle change.

When we put the focus of the day with the goals of the day, a change will hopefully result. That change is what will help us reach our sugar free lifestyle. Obviously, there is a lot to touch upon however, keeping it all organized will help in the success of it all.

To sum up this chapter, we have focused on getting ready to embark upon a sugar free lifestyle. This guide kicks off that lifestyle via a seven day sugar free challenge. Each day of the challenge will have goals, a focus, and a change.

Following the sugar free challenge is optional however, there may be parts of the challenge that can work for you as you go sugar free.

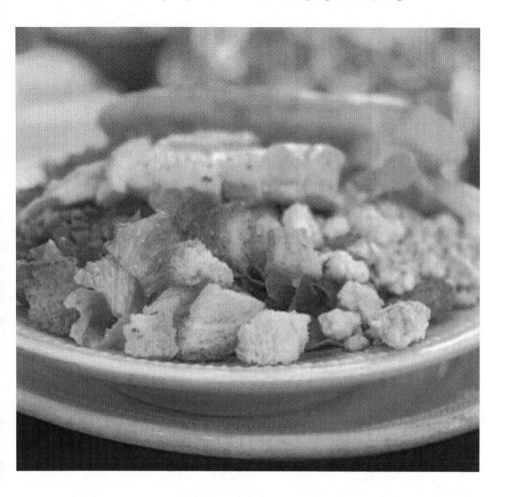

Day 1
What to expect that first day

Okay. So you have cleaned out the sugar from your kitchen cupboards and possibly gotten the sugar out of your system. Now we start the seven day journey.

The 'Big Goal of the Day' is to get started on the right track.

The first day is always the hardest it seems whenever we try something new. This is certainly no exception. Getting started on the right track means that we know what and how we are going to do this.

We know our triggers and we know the times of the day that we normally break for something to eat. It is often like clockwork that at noon we crave lunch. At four we need a snack.

Researchers say that we are essentially programmed or trained to expect food at certain times of the day. We are also triggered by the environment or where we are. So how do we deal with the sugar trigger?

The focus of day 1 is to deal with the sugar triggers.

As I have mentioned in the last chapter the focus is the psychological idea that we will focus on each day. Today we will focus on the triggers in the mind that make us hungry. In this journey, the triggers are related specifically to something sweet.

Here is my biggest daily hunger trigger.I am that person who is so hungry that I could eat everything in site at 4 pm every day. Why should I be so hungry every day at the same time?

There is a specialist says that I am hungry for food, especially sugar laden treats, at that time of the day for a reason. His theory has to do with my childhood. As a child I would come home from school and get a snack at that very time of the day. That snack was meant to be a positive reward that I would get for my hard work that day at school. It really makes sense-albeit in a Pavlovian kind of way.

You may share a similar trigger to my 4pm one. You may have a different one. The point is that we all have some kind of a hunger (sugary one probably) trigger at some time.

The biggest goal of the day is to identify the sugar craving triggers. The smaller goal is to deal with those sugar cravings.

In achieving the goals, the focus of the day is to think about those sugar craving triggers. How long have we been going through them? What time of the day do they usually occur? Where are we when it happens? w

 The change of that day resulting from those goals and focus ideas will therefore be to learn how to deal with our triggers.

Here is a worksheet for day 1:
Focusing on sugar craving triggers.

▸ **What time (s) of the day do the cravings occur?**

▸ **What are we doing when the cravings happen?**

▸ **How long have these daily cravings been going on?**

▸ **What event/events can the cravings be traced to?**

▸ **List three great ideas for dealing with the cravings tomorrow and forever:**
   1.

   2.

   3.

Here is how I dealt with my first day goals and focus.

My worksheet (also my focus for the day) looks something like this when it comes to (my big goal) dealing with my sugar craving triggers.

1. **Goal: Anticipate the cravings.**
   I learned to realize that my trigger time of the day will be occur daily. As a resultPlan ahead rather than hit 4:00 and realize that you are hungry.

2. **Goal: Have a plan.**
   I learned how to plan how I will deal with my sugar triggers. Here are some of my dealing ideas. Be so busy doing something that I would forget that it is 4:00. Have a sugar free snack waiting for me in anticipation. Just be one step ahead of the trigger.

3. **Goal: Take notes.**
   This is basically keeping a journal. This is a goal that I enacted for the entire week. From this day, in my journal I started to write down the time of day that my trigger hit, what I did

about it, and whether or not my action work for me.

4. **Plan for the next trigger.**
   This is where I added up my three goals and used them to plan for my future sugar cravings.

Day 1- The smaller goals of the day.

I just shared my big goal of the day and the smaller goals that were related with it. While dealing with my sugar triggers is important, there were a few smaller goals that I wanted to address on the first day.

For me, I wanted to face my beverage intake goals on that first day in addition to my crave triggers. As a result of addressing my beverage intake goal, I rediscovered water. There really are many benefits to drinking more water and I wanted to be part of that.

Not only is water sugar free, it also replacing something that is not. Water also helped me reach another smaller goal of keeping hydrated.

Here is how I made rediscovered water. I set a goal on how much water per day I would like to drink and how I will reach that goal. I found that water is a great way to 'detox' from drinking sugary drinks.

My water drinking goal was the suggested goal of many experts, eight 8 ounce glasses per day (64ounces or 1/2 gallon). I purchased an easy to carry tumbler which I use every day. By the way, there are water alternatives out there that some experts say are very similar to water.

To this day I like to make drinking water convenient. I have several reusable grab and go containers of water sitting in my refrigerator. Each is a convenient size and easy to carry or store with me while I am on the go.

To sum things up, the focus on this first day of giving up sugar was dealing with those sugar triggers. My goals had to do with identifying and dealing with my triggers as well as drinking more water. As a result of the day, I made a change in learning how to deal with my triggers. I also rediscovered drinking water.

Day 2
Dealing with my feelings.

There really is nothing like waking up on day two of anything knowing that you made it through day 1.

That is pretty much what I felt like when I woke up on day two of my sugar free challenge. It was very motivating for me to wake up on day two knowing that I had a successful day one.

My big goal of day two was to deal with my feelings and mind games.

My mind had a lot to do with the reasons why I decided to ditch the sugar in my life in the first place. I wanted my goal to be focusing on ditching the sugar and doing it without the self doubts that can be detrimental to any goal.

Those mind games can really sabotage any goals included a diet change. Getting in touch with my feeling helped me identify those mind games. The result would be knowing that they were just mind games and focusing my mind towards my goals.

Dealing with my mind games made be become more aware of what was going on in my mind. Most specifically for me was to become more aware of my feelings. If I were to be down on myself I knew that I would be more apt to rediscover sugar.

My focus for day two was to be aware of my feelings.

We all know that if we do not identify or deal with our feelings, something else can happen instead. For some folks that would be like eating our feelings.

So for me the big question was what was I thinking about when I was craving sugary treats. Was I angry at someone, sad about something, stressed, or even just board? My goal was to figure out what was going on in my head.

My big goal of the day was to figure out which of those feelings were related to my sugar cravings.

Smaller goals related to this big goal would be dealing with those feelings that lead to cravings. Journaling is one great way to both identify and deal with feelings.

Another goal could be to identify other ways to deal with the cravings. Other ways that have nothing to do with food. Like a hobby or some kind of exercise.

It may sound obvious to say, 'let's get in touch with our feelings' but really it can be a good thing to do. However finding the best way to do so can be a challenge in itself.

Documenting our feelings is a helpful way to get in touch with what we are thinking. So, let's somehow write this all down in a journal or in a notepad. Then we can keep track of how we are doing. Also, we can reference these feelings later on when we are looking for some motivation.

Here is a worksheet for day two.

▸ What am I craving and what time am I craving it?

▸ What was I thinking about before the craving popped into my mind?

▸ What was my emotional feeling at the time- happy sad, etc?

▸ How did I deal with that feeling?

Really all you need is a journal, pad of paper or a text file on your phone.

My change of the day was to learn how to deal with my feelings.

Once I learned how to identify my feelings and how they led to my craving sugar, I knew that the next step was to deal with the feelings.

I made a list of ten things that I could do instead of eating my feelings away with sugar. Here are some of the ideas that were on that list.

- Take a walk

- Drink a glass of water.

- Make a phone call.

- Check my email.

- Attack my laundry.

- Check out social media.

- Find something healthy to eat instead.

- Take a nap.

To sum things up, my focus on this day was to get in better touch with my feelings . My big goal was to identify those feelings that were more specific with my sugar cravings. My smaller goals were focused on identifying the mind games and finding other ways to deal with those feelings that would lead to my cravings. Another smaller goal it to keep positive in the mind.

Day 3
Getting into the groove

Yay! I managed to get through the two toughest days of giving up sugar. Now things are going to get easier!

My focus of the day is supporting my eating changes with one more thing.

Giving up sugar so far gave me some new found confidence. That confident feeling was a motivation that made me feel even more successful. It was time to do one more thing to aid in my success.

What else could I do to make my sugar free challenge even more successful? I could just follow my get rid of sugar in my life path. However, I want to do one more thing to make that path even better. Something new in my life would work perfectly here.

That made my biggest goal for the day to be identifying that one more thing. Technically, there certainly be a number of one more things that I could do to make my journey a successful one. I started with what I thought to be the more important thing I could incorporate into my daily life.

At this point in my week I was feeling pretty good about myself. Having one more successful goal achieved would make me feel even better about myself. There were several other goals I had been thinking about in addition to cutting out sugar.

My big goal of my third day was to actually do that one more thing to help me with my journey.

Not only did I identify that one more thing of upping up my physical game, I did it! Upping mu physical game had been a goal that I had in addition to cutting out sugar for a while. It just seemed like a good time for me to up my physical game at the same time.

I discovered the joy of walking. Walking not only helps control my weight and blood sugar, it also distracts me from those day one triggers.

I bought a fitness tracker and I love it. My tracker keeps track of my steps and other related things. However, what I like best about my fitness tracker is that it allows me to set personal goals. Meeting those goals makes me feel better about myself .

What will be your 'one more thing?

Walking may or may not be for you. However, you probably understand the idea behind one more thing. You may choose to take up yoga or bike riding instead. Or, maybe knitting or painting is your one more thing.

Here is the worksheet for day three of the sugar free challenge.

‣ Name one more thing that you could do to make your life better, in addition to the sugar free challenge.

‣ How will you go about doing this one more thing?

‣ What, if any, are the goals of your one more thing?

‣ List any additional ideas that you have for one more thing that you could do to better your life.

Let's sum up day three of this challenge.

My big goal of the day was to do one more thing to add to my success when it comes to giving up sugar. For me, that one more thing was to become more active.

That one more thing was directly related to my sugar free goal. However, your one more thing could be anything that you have been thinking of doing and doing it would help to bolster your confidence.

Smaller goals are also possible this third day of the sugar free challenge.

Within that one big goal of the day could be smaller goals. For me, in addition to upping my physical game, I had a smaller goal of walking a certain number of steps per day. Another smaller goal that I had was a goal of taking a work break to take a twenty minute walk per day.

Obviously, the focus of the day is one that one more thing. My focus was on becoming more active and doing so by walking.

My big change of the day is getting started with that 'one more thing'.

The big change that I wanted to make in my life as a result of this day was certainly to become more active. Part of my big change was telling myself to get off of the couch and walk. As a result, I started walking more . I also started keeping track of my walking.

I must admit that getting up and walking really did wonders for making me feel better about myself and my goals for the week. I also found that walking during my sugar craving time of the day helped me tackle the goals associated with day one as well.

Let me sum up the third day of my sugar free challenge. This was the day that I identified one more thing that I could do to better my life. For me, it was something that would help in my overall success with my sugar free challenge. Your one more thing could be something that helps in your success or something else that you have been thinking about doing.

In addition to identifying that one more thing, I actually acted upon it. For me. I identified that I wanted to up my physical game. As a result, I started to walk more. I even set goals as to how much and how often I would walk. I still do this today!

Day 4
The next thing that I did

By the time that I hit day four I had given up sugar, started drinking more water, and adopted a walking regimen.

This was the day to look beyond my weeklong challenge and think about next week and beyond. I was feeling good physically and mentally and decided that going without sugar was something that I wanted to continue to do.

The focus of the day is learning about the sugar in our food in order to continue on.

My day four was about learning about the sugar in my food. This quest for knowledge led to smaller goals such as learning the names of sugar and where sugar may be hidden in food.

While my big goal of the day was to think beyond this week, I had smaller goals as well.

There is more to learn about sugar that I once thought there was. Probably the most important thing to learn about sugar has to do with learning all of the different names for sugar. Once we know that names for sugar, we know what to look for when we read a food label

A smaller goal of the day was to learn how to read food labels. Learning how to read food labels led to other smaller goals such as learning about sugar alternatives.

I read up on the sugar alternatives that I could be using. This includes the natural alternatives as well as the manufactured alternatives. I used this knowledge to both write a manual for others to read and to publish recipes.

My big change of the day was to get into the habit of reading the labels on food before we eat them.

Learning how to read food labels was something that I had always wanted to do. As a result of this day, I would make reading food labels a habit.

We started out this day with a focus on what we will be doing beyond this week in order to maintain a sugar free lifestyle. Becoming more educated was the main goal with smaller goals within. The change that was made as a result was to make reading labels and other wanting to learn more about the sugar in the food that we eat.

To help you become more educate, and thus think about what is beyond this week, here is what I focused upon when I did my research.

1. What are the names of sugar?

2. What sugar is contained in the foods that I eat?

3. What alternatives could I be eating instead of the food with the sugar?

Day 5
Dealing with challenges

I remember years ago when I had joined a certain weight loss center that had clients attend weekly meetings. It was in those meetings that I was introduced to the 'saboteur'.

The 'saboteur' is that person in your life who may consciously, or unconsciously, try to sabotage your diet. Or in this case, your sugar free lifestyle.

This is the person who brings you ice cream and insists that you eat some since they went to all of that trouble to get it for you. Maybe that person is jealous of you or maybe they just don't want you to be successful.

The saboteur was indeed my biggest challenge. This was the well intended loved one who suddenly presented me with challenges to my goals. Sure, there were other challenges but, this was my biggest one.

My focus of the fifth day was dealing with challenges.

My focus was on the challenges that I perceived to be the stumbling blocks or obstacles that were presented to me during my sugar free challenge week. We seem to experience challenges on virtually every day of our lives.

While my saboteur was my biggest challenge, there certainly were smaller ones that I faced along the way. The 4 pm cravings from the first day of this challenge are just one of those daily challenges that are still with me today.

Since there are so many challenges it was best for me to start by making a list of the challenges. I then prioritized the list according to what I perceived to be the biggest challenges.

My next strategy was to conquer the challenges on my list. Of course, first I had to face each challenge before I could attempt to conquer them.

The focus of my day three was dealing with the challenges. My goal was first to identify those challenges. Identifying my challenges made my big change of the day obvious. The big change of my day would be making the changes that I needed to make making a plan for dealing with my challenges.

There were three steps to making my list of challenges. The first step was to list all of my perceived challenges. Next, I placed those challenges in order of importance as defined by the challenges that I perceived to be my biggest challenges.

The final step would be to cross of the list any challenge that after review I felt may really not have been a challenge and more of a concern and the challenges that I had really no control over.

One way to get started with our focus is to make a list of challenges.

Here is the worksheet of the day.

‣ Make a list of challenges.

1

2

3

4

5

6

‣ Now put those challenges in order of importance.

1

2

3

4

5

6

‣ Next cross off the list any challenge that may not really be a challenge or may be beyond control.

1

2

3

4

5

6

‣ Finally, for each challenge, plan an action.

1

2

3

4

5

6

Here is what my final list looked like.

1. Saboteur- say thanks but no thanks.

2. 4 pm cravings- take a 30 minute walk at 3:55.

3. Dessert pot luck with friends- bring something that has no added sugar and eat that.

4. Dessert after dinner with family- fill up on water first.

5. Sweet treats- find or make my own sugar free treats.

6. Alcohol- stick to the non sugary beverages.

Perhaps you would like to focus on just one challenge. That would be the one challenge that you anticipate to be the biggest. In my case that would have been the saboteur.

I really found that the entire process of identifying the challenges, narrowing them down, and making a plan of action was certainly very helpful. The process helped me stay away from sugar and get through the rest of the week.

To sum things up, the focus of the day was on the challenges that I perceived to be potential obstacles. My goal was to identify the challenges and rank them according to importance. My change of the day was to do something to deal with those challenges .

Day 6
Okay... I got this..but..

This was the moment of my weeklong challenge where, for a moment, I was thinking about the possibility of falling off the wagon.

Falling off the wagon, aka cheating, is something that runs through the mind of most anyone trying to make a change in their life. For me it was on day six.

My focus of the day was on 'falling of the wagon'

The idea of falling off the wagon reminds me of day five when I dealt with challenges. That is probably because the idea of falling off the wagon is indeed a challenge. What I think makes this day a bit different from yesterdays stumbling block challenge is that the sixth day is so much closer to the seventh day.

It is a good thing that we are human and as being humans, we do make mistakes every now and then. If my mistake was small and only a one time thing, I would probably just move on. After-all, the mistake could be as simply be one time hiccup.

I would consider falling off the wagon to be pretty much giving up on challenge itself as a whole. Cheating on the other hand, may be sneaking in a breath mint. I would have no intention of quitting over a breath mint and actually I would have so much guilt that I would never eat one again.

However, if I had hit the dessert bar at full throttle, my falling off the wagon could be something else.

It was on that day six that I had to remind myself of the journey that I had embarked upon during that week. My successes for the week were also something to be proud of.

To make a long story short, no, I did not fall off the wagon on day six or any other day of my challenge. In reality, I had gained so much confidence from that challenge that I was in it to win it. I would not let myself down for a breath mint.

As a result, I decided to make my goal of the day to focus on the future of my sugar free lifestyle rather than losing the battle on the sixth day.

The goal of the day is to list the reasons why I would stick to my sugar free lifestyle rather than fall off the wagon. There really were no smaller goals.

My change of the day was deciding how I would live my sugar free lifestyle. Sure, I had many ideas of how to do this before day six. However, I focused my thoughts for today on how to life my sugar free lifestyle rather than falling off the wagon and quitting.

Quitting the sugar free lifestyle seemed to be so much easier that adopting it. However, quitting would not solve anything in the end.

Day 7
This is how I feel now...

Yay! I made it to day seven of giving up sugar. To be honest, the week went by faster than I thought it would. It was not all that hard to do as well.

I was feeling pretty confident and like I wanted to continue on with this journey.

Here is how I felt after my seventh day without sugar.

After seven days of living without the added sugar I felt amazing. I had great energy, I was sleeping well, and I even lost a couple of pounds. I was feeling rather confident thanks to my success.

My success got me thinking about the next part of my journey. The next part of my journey would be making a life without added sugar in it my new lifestyle. While a totally sugar free lifestyle would be nice, I do like to eat fruit and fruit does have natural sugar in it.

My focus of the day was to think about how I felt after going without sugar for the week. I had made it through six days of focusing, goal setting and changes.

My biggest goal for the day was to accept my success. I found it to be important to also have a goal of the day to accept the success of the week and then to reward myself as needed. You could certainly praise yourself and brag as needed too.

You may expect that the big change of the day is to decide if this sugar free challenge, or a variation of it, is worth adopting as a lifestyle.

To sum things up, the focus of the day was to focus on the success of the week without sugar. My goal of the day was to accept my successes. My big change of the day was to decide whether I should make this a lifestyle change in the future.

Section 3-Living Your Sugar Free Life.

Forever sugar free.

After taking on a week of no sugar I must admit that I was feeling pretty good. I felt good both mentally and physically. To be honest I really liked that feeling too!

For me, feeling good was almost immediate after giving up sugar. I felt good after the first day of the sugar free challenge.

Going without sugar gave me plenty of energy without the highs and lows that I had been use to in the past from sugar. For me, this was my reward or measure of the success of my new lifestyle.

If you made it through the seven day sugar free challenge then you may be thinking about what comes next. Perhaps that means living a sugar free lifestyle for a longer period of time. For me, that would be forever.

However, you may feel as if simply cutting back on your total sugar intake is what works back for you. If cutting back on sugar is what works for you then you then you the sugar free challenge was probably of help to you as well.

Cutting back on sugar intake or omitting it entirely, means learning about sugar. We learn the names for sugar, how we are eating sugar, and how much sugar we are actually eating. Then we decide how we are going to get rid of the sugar or find substitutes for it.

We have already discussed how the average amount of sugar that the average person consumed shot up dramatically with the onset of convenience foods and the ease of purchasing those foods.

The big surprise of course is just how much sugar was going into food that we eat and do not even know about. This is why we learn the different names for sugar and how to read labels. Because we want to know the sugar that is added to the food that we buy and how much of it is in there.

Learning how to use alternatives for sugar is important too. Much of my sugar free life has been focused on switching over to sugar free alternatives for whatever I can do so for. I bake sugar free as a result and have switched over to sugar free beverage options.

I have noticed that over time I have become more of aware of sugar when it does cross my path. This may be happening for you too. It reminds me of when you go on a sodium free diet and then eat something salty. You certainly taste that salty food item with a vengeance .

Getting back to living your sugar free life. Finding what works best for you is important and will take some trial and error. It is also just as important to give yourself a break every now and then when needed.

I find that I have to do what works best for me. That means being as sugar free as possible or using alternatives when I can. It also means eating food with natural sugar, such as fruit. And, eating these naturally sweetened foods in moderation as they still can affect my blood sugar.

Tips for living a life with low or no sugar.

Here are a few more tips that may be of some help to you. If you know that you need coffee and you enjoy it with your specific sweetener, carry additional packets with you or have them readily available where you may need them.

Heading to a restaurant may mean dessert or beverages that contain sugar. Obviously, stick to the water or sugar free beverages. Even a glass of wine is better than that sugar laden margarita.

Order that dessert if you really have to and then eat a bite of it and give it to someone else or place a napkin over it. Even better, study the many before you head on out to the restaurant to plan out your order before you even get there.

What about parties and gatherings? If you can, bring a dessert that does not contain a lot of sugar. Even fresh fruit is a good option. And stick to the water based or sugar free beverages.

I must say that after years of avoiding sugar, a lot of it looks disgusting to me now. I am talking about the processed candy and baked desserts that have just too much of everything in them. No longer do I find those appealing. This could happen to you too!

My Sugar Free Thoughts

Best tips for expectations and success

This is where I share some final thoughts with you.

My tips are intended to give some inspiration and in a way, camaraderie. After all, we are all in some way survivors of sugar right?

Keep in mind that not everything works for everyone, I want to share some ideas that have worked for me. Take from this what works best for you.

My tips are simply the ideas and actions that worked for me.They may or may not work for you. In the end, they may simply serve as inspiration.

Later on in the book I have 120 ideas that you can do to go sugar free. In a way, those are tips too.

The tips here are what I would call my most important ones.

Tip 1- Keep the sugar out of the kitchen.

If you followed the sugar free challenge, you probably have already cleaned out your kitchen. The next thing to do is to think about keeping the sugar our of the kitchen.

You could easily decide to never buy the sugar laden products and know that they are not coming into your kitchen But, you still need to deal with other ways the sugar will get into your house.

Tip 2- Be prepared for temptations.

Temptations happen every day and when it comes to sugar, there is no exception. I find that I am more successful when I walk into the situation prepared for the possibility of temptation and with a plan on conquering it.

Tip 3- Decide whether you will be totally sugar free or sugar limited.

I decided that for the short term, I would cut out all sugar. Then, as I got better at controlling sugar, I would bring back fruit in moderation. I love fresh fruit and the benefits from eating it. In comparison to other foods that we eat that also contain sugar, most fruit is not so bad especially in moderation.

Tip 4-Make a meal plan for the week and then shop by it.

Here is the irony. I have never been good at making a meal plan . However, I do have friends who swear by making menu plans in advance . They will then make a shopping list according to their menu plans.

Making a shopping list also helps them keep on track with their food and budget. The meal plan idea is a really good idea because it helps you keep organized and in control of both your meals and your budget.

Meal plans are usually made at the beginning of the week or a week a head of time. They are helpful in organizing the food that you purchases. For example, if you were to plan two meals that call for chicken you can buy enough chicken for both of those meals. Or you could use the leftovers from one meal to use in the other.

By using a meal plan, you can plan out a shopping list. While you will add your meal plan food to your list, you can also include into your list foods that you may want to introduce into your diet. Specifically, the food that will replace your sugar and sugar laden food.

Tip 5- Always remind yourself about why are you cutting out sugar.

What actually brought you here or what needs to be fixed. Your reasons for cutting out sugar are your goals. You may also have smaller goals along the way too.

For example, you may be cutting out sugar for health reasons. While the main goal may be to lose weight, a smaller goal may be to become a smarter shopper. Another smaller goal may be to learn how to bake with alternative sweeteners.

Tip 6-Write down your goals, If you haven't done so yet.

Write down your goals. Make a copy if you need to to post on your refrigerator or desktop if you need motivation. Then write down how you will measure your success for meeting your goals.

Writing down your goals is a great motivator to keep you focused. Sometimes, there could be a reward for meeting goals as well.

Tip 7- Recruit a buddy.

You do not necessarily need to recruit a buddy to go sugar free. However, you could recruit someone to take walks with or go to the gym with.

I have a couple of recruited buddies that I walk with three days a week. One of those buddies became an on again off again sugar avoided too.

While I may have recruited my buddies to keep me walking, something even better evolved from it. Talking to my buddies while we walk has been incredible therapy for both myself and by buddies. Talking out my worries helps me stay away from sugar and other snacks by the way.

Those are some of my most important tips. Now I will share some smaller tips that may be of help too.

Here are some other tips that may help you plan your path:

- Keep a journal or diary.

- Add fitness or more fitness to your day.

- Eat a piece of fruit daily if you are craving sugar.

- Read and evaluate restaurant menus before you actually go there to determine what to order.

- Find new places to shop for groceries or order food from that may be better suited for your needs.

- Leave motivation pictures or words of wisdom posted on the refrigerator or on your desk to keep you motivated.

- Find someone to do this with you.

- Seek professional consultation from a registered dietician, physician, therapist.

•Subscribe to a magazine or newsletter that focuses on healthier eating.

•Follow social media accounts associated with your goals.

•A lesson that I learned was to not compensate for low sugar by adding something else, such as high sodium foods.

•Eat less of or avoid certain sugar alternatives that may cause a reaction. A good way to learn about reactions is to read the label or do your research online.

•Get use to reading labels on everything. Look for the many names of sugar and how much is in there.

• Find lower sugar alternatives to your usual food. My example would be discovering low fat Greek yogurt. My yogurt has no added sugar and it is high in protein.

•Get educated on sugar. Learn the names of sugar and which sugars may be better than others for you.

•Also, get educated on the many different sugar alternatives and which ones may be best for you.

•Plan out how you will stay on track in the longterm.

The tip that I have just mentioned are some of my favorite tips to share. There are more tips and strategies later on in this guide.

How to read a food label.

Learning how to read a food label is really essential for anyone who is thinking about what they are eating.

Nutrition Facts
Frozen Greek Yogurt Blueberry Treats

Amount Per Serving (1 g)

Calories 106

	% Daily Value*
Cholesterol 5mg	2%
Sodium 36mg	2%
Potassium 197mg	6%
Total Carbohydrates 15g	5%
Dietary Fiber 1g	4%
Sugars 11g	
Protein 10g	20%
Vitamin A	0.8%
Vitamin C	8.7%
Calcium	11.4%
Iron	1.5%

* Percent Daily Values are based on a 2000 calorie diet.

If you have never read a food label before, you may be surprised at what you will learn when you do read one. Remember, food labels are on packages because they contain important information for us.

By law, in the USA, there needs to be a food label on the food that we purchase at the local grocery store. Certainly, we must assume that there is a reason for that law.

There is actually more than one important label on food that we need to read.

The first label is the label that tells us about the nutrients and servings in the food. The second label tells us about the ingredients via a listing.

Here is what is important to read in the first, nutrient and serving label when it comes to our goals.

- Serving Size
- Servings Per Container
- Calories
- Total and Added Sugars

Also worth noting in this nutritional label are sodium, fat, cholesterol, protein, and percentages of nutrients.

Here is what else is important on that label.

Obviously, noting the added sugar in the food that we eat is important. However, it is really important to note the serving sizes and servings per container. A can of sugared soda may seem like the amount of added sugar may not be that high however, upon further inspection, that can may hold as much as two servings in it. That would certainly double the amount of sugar consumed than you had originally thought if you were to drink the entire can.

While calories and sugars are important to me, I would say my biggest shock usually comes from the serving sizes. Start noting servings sizes especially on what you may be thinking is an individual sized product.

Then there is the ingredient label.

This is often the label with words that you cannot pronounce or define. Most importantly, this is the label that tells you the ingredients, listed by importance, that are added to your food.

The ingredient label tells us more specific information about the sugar that is in our food. Certainly, naturally added sugar, like that from fruit for example, may not be a bad thing. However, that naturally added sugar may also be accompanied by additional added sugar in order to make something taste more palatable.

Here is what the FDA says about added sugar:

> **The definition of added sugars includes sugars that are either added during the processing of foods, or are packaged as such, and include sugars (free, mono- and disaccharides), sugars from syrups and honey,**

and sugars from concentrated fruit or vegetable juices that are in excess of what would be expected from the same volume of 100 percent fruit or vegetable juice of the same type. The definition excludes fruit or vegetable juice concentrated from 100 percent fruit juice that is sold to consumers (e.g. frozen 100 percent fruit juice concentrate) as well as some sugars found in fruit and vegetable juices, jellies, jams, preserves, and fruit spreads

Every time that I read any food label I look for the following:

•Sugar ingredients in the product by their name.

•Where on the ingredient listing are those sugar ingredients (is sugar the first ingredient listed?)

•Total sugars in the product.

•How many servings are in the container.

•How much of the product constitutes a serving.

I have read so many labels over the years that reading the label is usually the first thing that I do when I am looking at food, beverages, and even medicine.

You may be just looking to limit the amount of sugar that is added to your diet. Or you may be looking to only consume natural sugar in your diet. A food label can help you identify these sugars in order for you to make your decisions.

In the last chapter of this manual you will find a listing of names of sugar. Hopefully, this list will help you with your food and sugar decisions.

Learning how to use sugar alternatives.

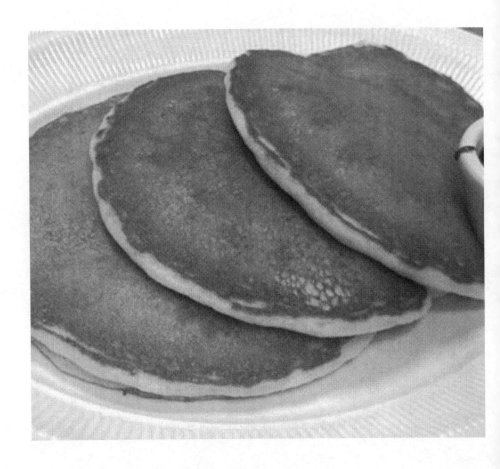

I have learned how to make and enjoy food and beverages with alternatives to sugar. Some sugar alternatives are better than others. This often has to do with what you are using the alternatives for.

If you have read my book about baking with sugar alternatives, then you know that there are many different kinds of sugar alternatives. Some sugar alternatives are better than others when it comes to baking while other alternatives are better at sweetening up what we are drinking.

Sugar is not just for sweetening.

What you should know is that sugar does more than just add sweetness to a recipe. Sugar also adds volume, and certain other baking properties too. These properties may or may not be replicated when we use an alternative to sugar. The properties really depend upon the alternative that we choose.

You can read more about using alternatives in recipes in my book 'Baking with Sugar Alternatives'. There are a lot of sugar alternatives available. If you are interested in using them in your kitchen then I recommend having more than one kind of sugar alternative around since some are better than others in certain situations.

My point is that if and when you are using sugar alternatives to the mixing bowl when you bake, you should know that you will need to compensate for more than just the sweet taste that you are replacing.

Depending on what you are baking, you will need to compensate for these properties. Use this knowledge for what you are baking for best results.

Sugar alternatives that you may want to have on hand.

A sugar free kitchen needs to take in consideration the various needs that a sugar alternative may have. You may be able to add the same kind of table sugar to beverages, baking, and as a topping on toast. However, the sugar alternative that is substituted in these scenarios may differ. Thus, you should have more than one kind of sugar alternative in your cupboard if you will be sweetening more than just your coffee.

Here is a shopping list for that sugar free cupboard.

If you are thinking about making a shopping list for you sugar free kitchen, here are some ideas that you may want to put on that list.

- Sugar alternatives for baking- I usually suggest a granular alternative that is 1:1 with sugar in volume. That means if you would use one cup of sugar in a recipe than one cup of the alternative would suffice. However, there are many varieties of these granular alternatives. For example, there are Splenda and Stevia granular alternatives. There are also granular blends that have sugar blended with a sugar alternative in them.

- Sugar alternatives for your coffee or tea. - Most folks are good with a packet of an alternative that is one serving that has already been prepared for you. While sometimes the packets may include the same granular products that you can use for baking, sometimes they will not. To clarify, the sweeteners that you may prefer to use to sweeten your coffee may not be suitable for baking with. Thus, you will need another sugar alternative for your beverages.

- Liquid sugar alternatives.-This is really for folks doing more than baking cookies or drinking tea. There may be occasions when you will need a liquid alternative. To be honest, I rarely use these however, I do have some in my cabinet.

- Natural sugar alternatives.-In the natural category of sugar alternatives that you would include in your cabinet, I would include sugar alternatives that you may or may not bake with. These are more of the 'healthier' options that you may use in place of sugar. For example, honey on toast instead of sugar. Other options may include molasses, agave or syrup. These are all dicey for recipes as they can taste sweeter than sugar and react differently to heat. I have made bread with honey and it turned out good!

Let's talk about sugar alternatives that may be in food that may already have been prepared for you.

You may have been purchasing these items with sugar in them in the past and now may want to replace them with a lower in sugar or sugar free item instead.

- Basic condiments. Ketchup is one condiment that usually has sugar added to it. However, there are lower sugar ketchup options available. I even have a recipe posted for a sugar free ketchup. Basic mustard, on the other hand, is usually made without sugar.

- Salad dressings, sauces, jams and jellies. If you really want to be sugar free, you could easily learn how to make these yourself. I have plenty of recipes on my site that you can refer to. Finding these items already prepared sugar free or low in sugar can be a challenge although, possible to do.

- Peanut butter, ice cream and other snacks. Peanut butter is available without added sugar or can be easily be made without sugar. The same goes for ice cream and snacks. I have a lot of recipes for these on my site.

- Replacing the other sugar items that you have. There is sugar in medicine, breath mints, and chewing gum. Now is the time to look for alternatives that may be sugar free or lower in sugar.

This is a good time to think about other changes that you may to make in your food purchases.

- New foods that you may want to start eating. This is where you can put fruits, vegetables, or even low carb or low fat foods.

- Your new go-to foods. If you were someone who had to have a chocolate bar every day and don't want to give that up then look for a chocolate bar that does not have all of that sugar added to it.

- Lastly, the beverages that you buy. We know that there can be hidden sugar in what we drink. This is a time to read the labels on fruit juices, soda, and even alcoholic beverages looking for that sugar.

How to Deal With Temptation

This is how I deal with sweet temptations.

Temptation is something that we touched on in our sugar free challenge It is not unusual for us to face temptation. We all know that there can be temptations in life every day.

As sugar survivors, we can become experts when it comes to facing those sugar temptations. Living in a sugar free world can be as easy or as hard as we make it to be.

You would think that once you learn how to shop, cook, and eat sugar free the rest just falls into place. For the most part, this is how it works out. However, there will always be some kind of temptation coming at you and usually it will happen when you least expect it.

Life is full of temptations and tests. We learn from these temptations and tests whether or not we beat them. What is perhaps important is that we are aware of them and that we are facing them

Here are my sugar temptations.

As humans, we face temptations all of the time. I think the easiest way to share with you how I deal with temptation is to simply list my temptations and then how I deal with them You probably share the same or similar temptations as well.

Chocolate.

Seriously, who doesn't crave a bit of chocolate at some time or another?

That chocolate craving can be in the form of a candy bar, slice of cake, or even in a beverage such as hot chocolate. It is best to prepare for that chocolate craving. I have some chocolate on hand and waiting.

My cure for my chocolate craving is to have a bite or two of an unsweetened or sugar free chocolate bar. I take my time enjoying that bite and I leave at least a few minutes between bites. This has taught me to enjoy and respect the pure taste of chocolate.

I suppose if I did not get that chocolate craving out of the way as soon as possible, it would haunt me for the rest of the day. I would then have to eat something else that I didn't even want to eat in order to distract me. So, I figure that just getting the craving out of the way early allows me to move on.

Baked Goods.

The worst for me is when I am at a celebration, such as a wedding or birthday, or when someone brings in something to share with others at work.

There really are just four options to choose from when it comes to dealing with the temptation of baked goods. The first option is to just go for it and eat the baked good. Of course, the result of that sugar can be really feeling bad about eating that sugar both physically and mentally.

The second option is to just not eat that baked good. Sometimes, you really may not be craving this food but, you want some because it is just sitting there looking at you. You may be surprised that this could be the easiest temptation to walk away from. Because if you are no craving it, not having any may not bother you after a while of not having it. You could just have a bite and through the rest away but, there is always that risk of having to eat more.

However, the third alternative is for those times when you just cannot say no. This does not happen every day and I would personally limit it to weddings and similar occasions. I will take a bite or two, not necessarily with the frosting since that is really no longer appealing to me (reformed frosting addict too...).

Then I will use this popular diet strategy. Take a bite or two of that cake, or whatever, and then sabotage the rest. Pour pepper over the rest of the cake, accidentally drop it on the floor (and clean it up), or just get rid of it before you finish it. The result is that you had your cake and you are still on track.

Lastly, you can learn how to make those baked goods yourself.

I learned how to bake sugar free. When I want cookies or a cake, for myself or to share, I can make it without the sugar. You can still enjoy the baked goods when you bake them yourself.

Beverages.

To be honest, being almost force-fed those sugary beverages as a kid kind of cured me of punches and the like. And because I have been sugar free for so long, I usually know when sugar in the form of a beverage has crossed my teeth.

My beverage temptation is from those alcoholic beverages.

I would not call myself a big drinker. It is usually wine in my case. However, every now and then I need something like a margarita. And, those pre-made ones or the pretty ones that you see in restaurants that cost as much as the meal, are sugar laden. Finding a low or no sugar alternatives was something that I had to do and that I did.

120 Things to Do to Go Sugar Free

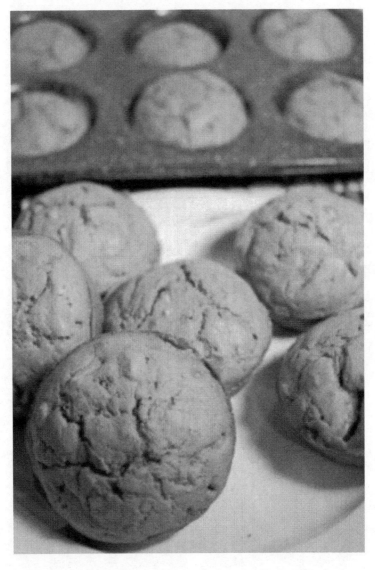

Ideas that help us get this going..

We discussed sugar, giving up sugar, adoption a sugar free lifestyle and dealing with temptations. Now we will explore more of my favorite tips to help motivate us all to success.

Keep this in mind.

I thought that making a list of what to do to go sugar free would be easier to follow than giving lengthy instructions on how to cut sugar out. The truth is that going sugar free **totally** is a lot different from cutting down on sugar and even more different from cutting out refined sugar.

Obviously, this whole cutting down on sugar intake is a personal thing as we are all motivated by our own reasons. However, we do have one thing in common. That common thread between us would be the need to reexamine sugar in our life.

Having said that, I would like to say that the first step, after deciding that there will indeed be a change, is to decide why you are making the change. After that you should decide what your goals are- or the end result of you cutting out sugar. Also, will this be a short-term temporary thing or a lifetime change for you?

Here are 120 ideas of things that you can do to go sugar free.

Some of these ideas may seem familiar to you. Others may be reminders. All are simply ideas that may or may not inspire something in your journey.

1.   See a medical professional for advice on whether or not you should be cutting out sugar from your diet. This is usually recommended when you are making a change in your diet.

2.   Write down what you are consuming in an average day. Keep a journal and don't adjust your eating. Be honest and write everything down. Do this for more than one day to get an accurate

reading. A full week of journal keeping, including a weekend, may offer a good insight for you.

3. Go through that journal and identify the sugar that you consumed that could have been avoided. Those extra cookies, fancy coffees, and ice cream for example. Separate this list between natural sugars, such as those that came from fruit, and the processed sugars (soda, candy etc).

4. Now go through that journal again. Identify the sugar that could have been a sugar alternative. The office coffee for example. that could have used a 'green packet' rather than the 'white packet'.

5.   Identifying the sugar in your journal can be confusing. This is a good time to become acquainted with the sugars. You can find a listing of the names here https://www.choosemyplate.gov/what-are-added-sugars

6.   Decide what your goals are. Are you cutting back on sugar to control your intake for example? Are you pre-diabetic? Or perhaps you simply want to lose weight. Many people simply want to cut back on the amount of sugar that they eat in a day. Experts suggest that the average American should consume about 10% of their

calories from sugar. For a 2000 calories a day diet, that would be about 200 calories should come from sugar. Again, this may not be for everyone as a medical professional will advice what is best for you.

7.   Going back to that journal, are your food groups balanced? That is, sometimes lacking in one area can lead to cravings in another area. You can learn more about food groups here https://health.gov/dietaryguidelines/2015/ guidelines/chapter-1/a-closer-look-inside-healthy-eating-patterns/#food-group

8.   Also, portions can be an important thing to know as well. You may be thinking that you are okay with the natural sugar since you had a natural fruit juice and an apple. However, some juices may have more than one serving in an average cup or some apples may be larger than others. This portion issue can lead to consuming more sugar than you may have intended to consume. Read about it here https://health.gov/ dietaryguidelines/2015/guidelines/chapter-1/a-closer-look-inside-healthy-eating-patterns/#fruits

9.   You may be someone who wants to cut out all added sugar. Maybe the controlling the

sugar was not your thing. This is where you should decide which path is for you.

10. Get yourself ready for your change. Psych yourself up, motivate yourself, and praise yourself for your change.

11. Clean out your sweet stash before you start. Just get rid of it to avoid any temptations that can come your way. This includes a sugar stash in your kitchen, desk, or even your car.

12. Sometimes not telling everyone about your changes can be a good thing as some well-meaning folks do not help. Other times, having a support system can be of help. The point here is that this is a good time to think about how you will deal with the people in your life and your goals.

13. Keep a journal of what you are eating. This will help you identify what is working or where your week spots may be. Your journal can also help you learn when you are craving sugar or how you are feeling as well.

14. Educate yourself on not only the names of all sugars, but the names of sugar alternatives

or sugars that you may want to include in your diet.

15. Also, learn about the physical effects and what is normal when you cut out sugar. Some effects may be normal while others may need medical interventions.

16. Sugar cravings, especially early on, can often be relieved by eating something that you may perceive as being sweet even though there really is no sugar in it.

17. Cravings can be distracted by exercise such as just going for a walk.

18. It helps to have a list of ways to distract those cravings handy when you may need to reference it.

19. Keep your thoughts away from sugar by taking up a new hobby such as knitting, going for a walk, cleaning out a drawer, or getting as far as possible from the triggers of sugar cravings.

20. If you physical symptoms do not subside, certainly seek some medical advice.

21. Drink more water. It will keep you full and can often fulfill that hunger need or craving.

22. Learn how to cook and bake without adding sugar to your recipes.

23. Invest in healthier alternatives to sugar, such as raw or dried vegetables, snacking.

24. It can be easier to start a sugar restricted diet by first restricting the processed sugars first. Processed sugars are usually the ones added to cookies, soda, etc. Then as time goes on work on eliminating the other sugars.

25. Eating more of smaller meals rather than three large meals can help keep your blood sugar more stable.

26. Look for sugar in what you are purchasing. Become your own expert when it comes to reading a food label. I always read the labels on food before I buy something. I look for both the obvious added sugar, and the hidden sugar that may have been added.

27. While you may think that not a lot of sugar has been added in something, it is important to take in consideration the serving size. For example, a candy bar may seem like it has a small amount of sugar added to it when you read the label however, upon further examination

you may notice that there are more than one serving in that candy bar and thus, a lot more sugar than you may have thought. You can read more about food labels here https://www.fda.gov/Food/LabelingNutrition/ucm274593.htm

28.   Common side effects of giving up sugar, that is those effects that people mention the most, include: headaches, changes in mood, irritable, more happy, food cravings, feeling 'scatterbrained' or dizzy, fatigued, energized, headaches, sleepy, less sleepy, and/or more energetic.

29.   Not every side effect is felt by everyone who gives up sugar. Most side effects subside after a week or so. If yours do not subside or they just seem unusual, certainly seek a professional's advice.

30. Rethink your dining out strategy. If you feel comfortable with ordering the right food at the places your normally eat at, keep going there. However, if you are afraid of those sweet temptations that you once embraced, you may need a new strategy. For me, I just had to stay away from those places. Actually, learning how to cook and bake for myself using the ingredients

that I choose, solved a lot of that dining out temptation.

How to deal with temptation.

You cannot always avoid those temptations of sugar so you probably should learn how to deal with them if you want to be sugar free.

31. If it is in your home, get rid of it.

32. If it is on your plate, sabotage it by putting something unpleasant over it.

33. If someone has served it to you and you do not want to seem rude, take one small bite and put it out of site.

34. Take one bite and then spit it out (politely).

36. Craving sugar? Opt for a sugar free beverage instead, Water usually works for me.

37.   Keep a list of things that you can do rather than eat sweets. I keep a list of 5 minute, 10 minute, and 20 minute tasks that I need to get done but, always forger or cannot find time to do.

38. Start a penny or dollar jar and contribute to it whenever you taste or think about tasting sugar. Use the contents of the jar later on as a reward.

39. Like mom use to always say, have a piece of fruit or a carrot.

40. Some folks swear by the keeping a journal of feelings when you are craving something.

41. Chew gum.

42. Have a mint. I am a fan of popping a sugar free mint when I am thinking about something bigger and sweet. Mints seem to satisfy me and change the subject at the same time.

43. Eat a few sugar free chocolate chips rather than a candy bar.

44. Learn how to savor that taste if you allow yourself just one bite.

45. Allow yourself one bite and then get the remainder out of site.

46. Frozen chocolate is a lot harder to bite into than the room temperature stuff.

47. Walk. I am a sucker for those books on tape (which really aren't on tape any more) and a walk around the block or my backyard.

48. Find comfort with a pet. I am a dog person and have been diverted from disaster many a time thanks to my dogs.

49. Allow yourself a day, a weekend, or a meal off every now and then.

50. Forgive yourself. Dust yourself off and get back on the journey when you need to do so.

25 questions for you.

51. Identify the reason why you are giving up sugar. What was the straw that broke the camel's back?

52. What will the end result be of your sugar free plan be? Lose weight? Control blood sugar?

53. How long will you be cutting out sugar for? Is this a life change or temporary thing?

54. Do you plan on giving up all sugar?

55. Do you plan on just giving up refined sugar?

56. Will you learn about adding sugar alternatives to your life?

57. Seriously..is this a diet to lose weight are are you just happy to give up sugar?

58. How will you know if this is working for you? Will you have 'mile markers' along the way?

59. Have you consulted a doctor? You should especially if you are cutting out sugar for medical purposes.

60. Will you be introducing something new into your diet to distract you from the absence of sugar? Some folks like to increase their protein intake for example.

61. Have you done your research? By research, I mean have you investigated what will

happen to your body when it goes without sugar? Or the alternatives to sugar?

62. Who are you going to tell about this change? You friends? Family?

63. How do you plan to do with the short term effects of going without sugar?

64. Are you ready to get rid of everything that has sugar in it from your home?

65. Do you have a support system? The people who you can talk to when you may be tempted or needed some support.

66. How will you handle the surprise sugar that may come into your life? The cookies in the break room, the fancy coffee someone got for you, the piece of wedding cake that you were served?

67. Are you ready to learn how to read labels on every food that you are interested in?

68. Do you know what to look for on those labels?

69. So, what if you are tempted with a craving. What will you do?

70. List five five minute tasks that you can do instead of hitting the sugar.

71. List five 10 minute tasks that you can do instead of hitting the sugar.

72. List five 20 minute tasks that you can do instead of hitting the sugar.

73. How did you feel after the last time that you ate something sweet that you now regret eating?

74. What were you thinking about before you are that sweet treat?

75. What is your biggest piece of advice that you would like to give to yourself when you are feeling the need for sweets?

With that, I will now share with you my 50 tips on how to go sugar free.

Obviously, not everything will be suited or the best for you. However, if there is something that you can gain from these tips, that will be a positive motivator for you.

76. Go see your doctor and make sure that giving up sugar is good for you.

77.   See a nutritionist or dietician for assistance on your idea.

78.   Set a goal(s). Identify the purpose or what will be the result of giving up sugar.

79.   Decide if you will be giving up all sugar, some sugar, or just refined sugar.

80.   Consider having a last hoorah- that is your last cookie or whatever before you move on. For some folks saying goodbye works as motivation.

81.   Research your sugar. Learn the names of the sugar(s) you are wanting to get rid of.

82.   Research the alternatives to those sugars.

83.   Clean out the sugars from your life. Get rid of the cookies and other temptations.

84.   Map out how you will measure your progress.

85.   Decide how long you will be sugar free or if this will be a life-long change for you.

86.   For me, giving up sugar was a cold-turkey life change. I felt it would be easier to not

even have to think about sugar if I just gave up all sugar.

87.   Going from refined sugar to natural sugar (fruit for example) is a good way to transition to the sugar free world and fight off the sugar cravings at the same time.

88.   This is a great time to keep up that hydration. If you are not drinking your water, this could be a good time to start. Plus, how many times have you thought that you were hungry only to realize that you were just thirsty?

89.   Read those food labels especially with those foods that say they are low fat or low something else. Sometimes, they have to compensate for the loss of taste with adding additional sugar to the recipe.

90.   Other food that may surprise you with sugar include; crackers, yogurt, condiments, sauces, spice blends, juices

91.   Granola and trial mixes often have sugar added to them.

92.   If a fruit juice says 'cocktail' or 'blend' on the label it may have sugar added to it as well.

93.   On the other hand, if the label on cookies or something similar says that it is sugar free, it may be high in something else that you are avoiding, such as fat.

94.   Learning how to make your own ketchup or sauce is a helpful way to get through barbecue season.

95.   Possibly the worst sugar offender , according to the experts, are those sweetened beverages. Luckily, we are seeing more and more alternatives pop up in the market.

96.   Having said that, there are some water products out there that do have sugar added to them.

97.   Protein products, such as powders and bars, are sometimes sweetened with sugar to make them taste better.

98.   Most any kind of drink mixer has sugar added to it. Learn how to make your own mixer, explore other beverage options, or look for the 'skinny' options.

99.   Look for canned foods that are packed in their own juice or water rather than the usual stuff that has sugar products added to them.

100.   The same thing goes for the frozen bags of fruit. Opt for the fruit that has nothing added to it before it has been frozen.

101.   Learn how to freeze your own fresh produce so that you can control what goes into it.

102.   Dehydrating fresh fruit and vegetables is a great way to preserve and also make good food for snacking on.

103.   Relax. You can still enjoy those peanut butter and jelly sandwiches. Make your own peanut butter and jelly without the sugar added to them or buy some already made for you.

104.   Sure, sugar free candy can help fill a void or craving but, eating too much of it in one sitting can prove to be irritating to the gastrointestinal system thanks for certain sweeteners that are used. I am somewhat an expert on this and would advise most folks to eat 'sugar free candy' in moderations.

105.   Just because it is a 'natural' sugar alternative does not mean that there is no sugar in

it. Not only do many of these have sugar in them, some have even more sugar that processed sugar per tablespoon.   106.   Baking or cooking with alternatives can be done. However, there usually are some modifications that must be made to the recipe as a result. I wrote a book on this topic.

107.   Those blended fruit smoothies that are suppose to be healthy for us may also be over-kill in the sugar department. Not only will they have the sugar from the fruit in them, they may also have sugar from other ingredients added to them such as honey or sugar itself.

108.   I once saw a recipe for a 'sugar free' copycat cereal-like candy bar. What was the first ingredient in it? Regular cereal. Thus, the recipe was not entirely sugar free.

109.   Just because a recipe says that it is 'sugar free' it may not be thanks to some of the ingredients that are added to it.

110.   Also, even the blandest of the cereals out there may have sugar in it.

111.   Obviously, you probably have already have heard that those fancy coffees out there are often laden with sugar.

112.   Added sugar are those sugars that are added to the products and recipes that we consume. Sometimes, an added sugar may not be a processed sugar even though it is an added sugar. An example of this would be molasses which can be used to sweeten a recipe but, is also a sugar.

113.   Glucose sugar is actually needed by the body to help nourish our blood cells and thus, our bodies. We need glucose for energy.

114.   Having too much or too little glucose in the blood can cause issues such as diabetes.

115.   Each gram of sugar contains 4 calories in it.

116.   The Dietary Guidelines for Americans recommends consuming less than 10% of calories per day from added sugars.

117.   The average American consumes more than 13% of total calories (or almost 270 calories) per day from added sugars.

Where to find sugar
Or how to know it is there.

This chapter is for what to look for on food labels.

The many names for sugar.

If you are avoiding eating sugar, you may want to get familiar with these names for sugars.

- Anhydrous Dextrose

- Confectioners or Powdered Sugar

- Dextrose

- Fructose

- Granulated Sugar

- Syrup

- Sucrose

- Nectar

- Maltose

- Brown Sugar

- Corn Syrup

- High Fructose Corn Syrup

- Honey

- Malt Syrup

- Molasses

- Raw Sugar

- White Sugar

- Invert Sugar

What is in my kitchen now
My sugar free shopping list

Earlier I discussed the sugar alternatives that I added to my cupboard when I went sugar free. Those items are always in my cabinet. I replace them as needed when I need to.

These items are what I will put on my shopping list. As I have mentioned, I do enjoy fruit in moderation. And ,fruit does come with its own natural sugar. This is something that I have decided to bring back into my life since going sugar free as apples do have many benefits from eating them.

I make my shopping list according to how I travel in the store. I start in the fresh product section and work my way around through dairy. I shop basically the perimeter of the store and then hit the aisles as needed

Fresh produce.

Always, I have lettuce (usually romaine), tomatoes (Roma) and various salad related items on hand at all times. Then there are the fruit choices.

MyPlate.gov suggests that most adults have between 1 1/2-2 cups in a day.

 I focus on the fruit that has low sugar and high benefits.

Avocados
Watermelon
Strawberries-
Lemons
Limes-
Apples (Granny Smith for example)-
Tomatoes-
Fruits that we think may be vegetables such as squash
Blueberries
Blackberries

For baking.

Earlier I shared the sugar alternatives that I have in my cupboard. I like to bake so I have plenty of sugar alternatives in my cupboard.

If you have read my sugar free baking guide then you know there is a lot that goes into using sugar alternatives while baking. This is especially true about the alternatives that are not natural because of their chemical composition.

My point is that because I like to bake a variety of foods, I have a variety of different kinds of sugar alternatives. When you bake with sugar, you have your granular white sugar, your brown sugar and probably a powdered variety.

When you bake with sugar free sugar, you may have more than just three kinds of sugar. Here are some sugar free alternatives that you may have. This list is adding to what we have discussed in earlier chapters.

The Natural Sugar Alternatives:

- Stevia (which is actually regarded as a GRAS and non-nutritive)

- Agave Nectar (as need for a recipe)

- Honey (local honey as needed).

- Molasses (as needed in for a recipe)

- Syrup (such as maple syrup, for recipe use)

- Coconut Palm Sugar (as needed)

- Sugar Alcohols (as needed for recipes)

The Artificial Sugar Alternatives:

- Sucralose

- Aspartame

- Saccharin (rarely on my list)

Sweet knowledge
Research, facts, and more

Where You Can Learn More

Start your research with these recommended sites in addition to visiting and signing up for the newsletter on https://thesugarfreediva.com .

Mayo Clinic -> http://www.mayoclinic.org/healthy-living/nutrition-and-healthy-eating/in-depth/artificial-sweeteners/art-20046936?pg=1 ->Artificial Sweeteners and Other Sugar Substitutes.

From MedilinePlus https://medlineplus.gov/ency/article/007492.htm

->Sweeteners - sugar substitutes

https://medlineplus.gov/druginfo/natural/682.html->Information on Stevia

U.S. Food and Drug Administration href="http://www.fda.gov/Food/IngredientsPackaging%20Labeling/FoodAdditives%20Ingredients/ucm397716.htm ->High-Intensity Sweeteners

Read about Saccharin https://www.fda.gov/Food/IngredientsPackagingLabeling/FoodAdditivesIngredients/ucm397725.htm#Saccharin

Learn about Aspartame https://www.fda.gov/Food/IngredientsPackagingLabeling/FoodAdditivesIngredients/ucm397725.htm#Aspartame

Read about Sucralose https://www.fda.gov/Food/IngredientsPackagingLabeling/FoodAdditivesIngredients/ucm397725.htm#Sucralose"

Find out about Steviol glycosides https://www.fda.gov/Food/IngredientsPackagingLabeling/

FoodAdditivesIngredients/
ucm397725.htm#Steviol_glycosides

https://thesugarfreediva.com/how-to-measure-
sugar-alternatives/

https://thesugarfreediva.com/use-high-intensity-
sweeteners/

In conclusion
Living a sugar free lifestyle ...forever?

Maybe you are doing this because you were told that you have to. Maybe you are wanting to control the sugar in your life. OR it could be that you want to lose a few pounds and you feel that this is how you can do it.

My journey is about controlling sugar rather than sugar controlling me.

This is an ongoing journey and something that I deal with on a daily basis. However, over time it has become easier for me to control the sugar in my life.

As a result of controlling the sugar in my life, I feel better both mentally and physically,

What happens in your journey is certainly up to you. I can only share with you what has worked for me along with a few other ideas

Are you breaking up with sugar?

Please visit me on thesugarfreediva.com and leave me a message letting me know how it is going for you.

You can also visit me on Facebook-

https://www.facebook.com/thesugarfreediva/

Pinterest-

https://www.pinterest.com/thesugarfreediva

and Instagram.

http://instagram.com/thesugarfreediva

Made in the USA
Lexington, KY
20 April 2019